Pure Carnivore

Simplify Your Diet, Amplify Your Health with Meat-only Diet

Sharon Byers

Copyright © 2024 by Sharon Byers

Disclaimer

The information presented in this book is for educational and informational purposes only and should not be construed as medical advice or a substitute for professional healthcare. Always seek the guidance of your physician or other qualified health provider with any questions you may have regarding your health or a medical condition.

The author is not responsible for any adverse effects, losses, or damages that may arise from the application of information contained in this book. All individuals are encouraged to consult with a licensed healthcare provider before beginning any dietary, exercise, or lifestyle change program.

Results shared in this book are not guaranteed and may vary from individual to individual. The reader assumes full responsibility for their decisions and actions after reading this book.

Note: Dietary changes can have significant effects on your body, and any drastic dietary shifts should be undertaken cautiously and with professional guidance.

TABLE OF CONTENTS

Contents

Introduction

Embracing Simplicity: The Pure Carnivore Philosophy

In a world increasingly obsessed with complex diets and food trends, the allure of simplicity has never been stronger. The Pure Carnivore philosophy offers a return to basics, stripping away the confusion and chaos that often accompany modern eating habits. This approach is not just about reducing what you eat but about focusing on the most nutrient-dense, bioavailable foods available: animal products. Welcome to the Pure Carnivore lifestyle, where simplicity meets superior health.

The Case for Simplicity

Why choose a diet that revolves around simplicity? The answer lies in the myriad benefits that come from focusing on whole, unprocessed animal foods. In our quest for health, we often turn to intricate diets with countless rules, restrictions, and ingredients. These can be overwhelming, difficult to maintain, and ultimately ineffective. The Pure Carnivore approach cuts through this noise, offering a straightforward path to wellness that our ancestors instinctively followed.

Ancient Wisdom

The history of human nutrition is deeply rooted in animal-based diets. Our ancestors thrived on diets primarily composed of meat, fish, and other animal products. They hunted, gathered, and consumed what was available in their environment, and these nutrient-dense foods provided everything they needed for optimal health. By returning to this ancestral way of eating, we can tap into a wealth of nutritional wisdom that has stood the test of time.

Modern Health Benefits

The Pure Carnivore diet is not just a nostalgic nod to the past; it is a powerful tool for achieving and maintaining optimal health today. Numerous studies and countless personal testimonials highlight the benefits of a meat-only diet, from improved mental clarity and sustained energy to enhanced physical performance and robust immune function. This diet addresses many modern health issues caused by processed foods, excessive sugar, and empty carbohydrates.

What to Expect in This Book

"Pure Carnivore: Simplify Your Diet, Amplify Your Health" is designed to guide you through the principles and practices of the Pure Carnivore lifestyle. Each chapter delves into different aspects of this way of eating, providing comprehensive information, practical advice, and inspiring success stories. Whether you are new to the carnivore diet or looking to refine your approach, this book offers valuable insights and actionable steps to help you achieve your health goals.

A Roadmap to Success

We will begin with an exploration of the fundamental principles behind the Pure Carnivore philosophy. From there, we will delve into the nutritional science that supports this diet, explaining why animal products are uniquely suited to nourish our bodies. You will learn how to transition smoothly to a carnivore diet, including tips for meal planning, addressing common concerns, and overcoming potential challenges.

Real-Life Transformations

Throughout the book, you will encounter real-life stories of individuals who have transformed their health and lives through the Pure Carnivore diet. These testimonials provide tangible proof of the diet's effectiveness and serve as motivation for your own journey. Their experiences demonstrate that embracing simplicity can lead to profound changes in health, well-being, and overall quality of life.

Practical Guidance

We understand that adopting a new diet can be daunting, especially one as seemingly restrictive as the Pure Carnivore diet. That is why we include practical tips for navigating social situations, dining out, and maintaining long-term success. This book is designed to be a comprehensive resource, offering support and guidance every step of the way.

The Promise of Pure Carnivore

By embracing the Pure Carnivore lifestyle, you are choosing a path that prioritizes simplicity, nutrient density, and optimal health. This diet is not about deprivation or rigid rules but about nourishing your body with the foods it was designed to thrive on. The journey may challenge your preconceptions about nutrition, but it also promises unparalleled benefits.

Your Journey Begins

As you embark on this journey, remember that the Pure Carnivore diet is more than just a way of eating; it is a commitment to yourself and your health. It is an invitation to simplify your diet, amplify your health, and reclaim your well-being. Through the pages of this book, we will explore how returning to the basics can unlock a healthier, more vibrant life.

Welcome to the Pure Carnivore Revolution. Let's begin this transformative journey together, embracing simplicity and experiencing the profound health benefits of going back to basics.

Chapter 1

The Essence Of Simplicity

Why Simplifying Your Diet Matters

In today's fast-paced, information-saturated world, the concept of simplicity is often undervalued. We are bombarded with dietary advice, superfoods, supplements, and complex meal plans that promise optimal health. Yet, with all this complexity, many of us are left feeling overwhelmed, confused, and, paradoxically, less healthy. This chapter delves into why simplifying your diet is not just a refreshing approach but a necessary one for achieving lasting health and well-being.

The Complexity of Modern Diets

Overwhelm and Decision Fatigue

The modern diet landscape is characterized by an abundance of choices and conflicting information. This complexity can lead to decision fatigue, where the sheer number of options and decisions to be made regarding food choices can cause stress and poor decision-making. When you are constantly trying to navigate through a myriad of dietary rules and recommendations, it is easy to become overwhelmed and lose sight of the fundamental principles of good nutrition.

The Problem with Processed Foods

Processed foods, which dominate modern diets, are designed to be convenient and palatable. However, they often come at the cost of nutritional quality. These foods are typically high in refined carbohydrates, unhealthy fats, and artificial additives, contributing to various health issues, including obesity, diabetes, and heart disease. Moreover, the complexity of ingredients and additives in processed foods can lead to food sensitivities and inflammatory responses in the body.

The Case for Simplification

Nutrient Density and Bioavailability

The essence of a simplified diet lies in focusing on nutrient-dense, bioavailable foods. Animal-based foods, particularly those included in the Pure Carnivore diet, are rich sources of essential nutrients that are easily absorbed and utilized by the body. These include high-quality proteins, healthy fats, vitamins, and minerals that are crucial for optimal health. By simplifying your diet to include primarily animal products, you ensure that every bite you take is packed with nutrition, supporting your body's needs effectively.

Reducing Inflammation

Inflammation is at the root of many chronic diseases, and diet plays a significant role in either exacerbating or alleviating inflammation. The Pure Carnivore diet, by eliminating common dietary triggers such as grains, legumes, and processed foods, helps reduce systemic inflammation. This reduction in inflammation can lead to improvements in various health conditions, including autoimmune diseases, digestive disorders, and metabolic syndrome.

The Simplicity of the Carnivore Diet
Fewer Ingredients, Greater Impact

The Carnivore diet is characterized by its simplicity: it focuses on meat, fish, eggs, and animal fats. This minimalist approach not only simplifies meal planning and preparation but also makes it easier to avoid potential allergens and irritants commonly found in more complex diets. By limiting your food choices to high-quality animal products, you eliminate the need to scrutinize ingredient lists and navigate through the maze of modern dietary guidelines.

Consistency and Sustainability

One of the significant advantages of a simplified diet is its sustainability. When your diet consists of a few staple foods, it becomes easier to maintain consistency. This consistency is key to achieving long-term health benefits. Unlike diets that require meticulous tracking of macronutrients, calorie counting, or frequent meal replacements, the Carnivore diet's straightforward nature makes it easier to adhere to and integrate into daily life.

Psychological Benefits of Simplifying Your Diet

Reducing Stress and Anxiety

Food-related decisions can be a significant source of stress and anxiety for many people. The constant worry about making the "right" food choices, avoiding "bad" foods, and following complex dietary rules can take a toll on mental health. By simplifying your diet, you reduce the mental burden associated with eating. Knowing exactly what you can and cannot eat removes the guesswork and allows you to focus on enjoying your meals without guilt or anxiety.

Building a Healthy Relationship with Food

A simplified diet fosters a healthier relationship with food. Instead of viewing food as a source of stress or confusion, you begin to see it as a means of nourishment and healing. The Carnivore diet encourages mindful eating, where you pay attention to your body's hunger and satiety signals and develop an appreciation for the nutritional value of your food. This shift in perspective can lead to a more positive and balanced approach to eating.

Practical Steps to Simplify Your Diet

Eliminate Processed Foods

The first step towards simplifying your diet is to eliminate processed foods. These foods are often loaded with unhealthy additives, preservatives, and artificial ingredients that can harm your health. Focus instead on whole, unprocessed animal products that provide pure, unadulterated nutrition.

Focus on Quality

When following the Carnivore diet, quality matters. Choose high-quality, ethically sourced animal products. Grass-fed beef, pasture-raised poultry, wild-caught fish, and organic eggs are excellent choices. These options not only provide superior nutrition but also support sustainable and humane farming practices.

Plan Simple Meals

Meal planning on the Carnivore diet is straightforward. Base your meals around high-quality protein sources, such as steak, chicken, fish, and eggs. Add healthy fats, like butter, tallow, or ghee, for cooking and flavor. Keep your meals simple and repetitive if necessary, to reduce decision fatigue and streamline your eating habits.

Embracing the Pure Carnivore Lifestyle
Long-Term Benefits

The long-term benefits of simplifying your diet extend beyond physical health. By adopting the Pure Carnivore lifestyle, you create a sustainable, nourishing way of eating that supports your overall well-being. Over time, you will likely notice improvements in energy levels, mental clarity, physical performance, and immune function. These benefits are a testament to the power of simplicity in achieving and maintaining health.

Community and Support

Joining the growing community of Carnivore diet enthusiasts can provide valuable support and motivation. Online forums, social media groups, and local meetups offer opportunities to connect with others who share your commitment to the Pure Carnivore lifestyle. Sharing experiences, tips, and recipes can enhance your journey and help you stay motivated.

The essence of simplicity lies at the heart of the Pure Carnivore philosophy. By focusing on nutrient-dense, bioavailable animal products and eliminating the complexities of modern diets, you can achieve lasting health and well-being. Simplifying your diet not only reduces stress and decision fatigue but also fosters a healthier relationship with food. As you embark on this journey, remember that the benefits of simplicity are profound and far-reaching. Embrace the Pure Carnivore lifestyle and discover the transformative power of going back to basics.

Chapter 2

The Nutritional Power Of Meat

Understanding the Benefits of a Meat-Only Diet

The nutritional landscape is vast and often confusing, with countless foods and diets claiming to be the key to optimal health. Amidst this complexity, the Carnivore diet stands out for its simplicity and the undeniable nutritional power of meat. This chapter explores the myriad benefits of a meat-only diet, delving into the essential nutrients found in animal products and how they contribute to overall health and well-being.

The Nutritional Composition of Meat
High-Quality Protein

Protein is a critical macronutrient that plays a vital role in nearly every biological process. Meat, particularly red meat, is one of the best sources of high-quality protein. The amino acids in meat are complete, meaning they contain all nine essential amino acids that the body cannot produce on its own. These amino acids are crucial for muscle repair and growth, immune function, hormone production, and overall cellular health.

Healthy Fats

Contrary to outdated beliefs that fats are detrimental to health, the right types of fats are essential for bodily functions. Meat, especially fatty cuts, provides a balanced mix of saturated and unsaturated fats. These fats are vital for hormone production, brain health, and energy. Additionally, fats help with the absorption of fat-soluble vitamins (A, D, E, and K) found in meat.

Essential Vitamins and Minerals

Vitamin B12

Vitamin B12 is a crucial nutrient involved in red blood cell formation, nerve function, and DNA synthesis. It is primarily found in animal products, making meat an essential component of a diet for maintaining adequate B12 levels. Deficiency in this vitamin can lead to anemia, neurological issues, and cognitive impairments.

Iron

Iron is essential for transporting oxygen in the blood and supporting metabolic processes. Heme iron, the type found in meat, is more readily absorbed by the body compared to non-heme iron found in plant foods. Adequate iron intake helps prevent anemia and supports overall energy levels.

Zinc

Zinc is a vital mineral involved in immune function, wound healing, and DNA synthesis. Meat, particularly red meat and shellfish, is an excellent source of bioavailable zinc. This mineral supports the immune system, promotes healthy skin, and aids in cellular repair and regeneration.

Creatine

Creatine is a compound found almost exclusively in animal products. It plays a critical role in energy production, particularly in high-intensity exercise. Supplementing with creatine is common among athletes, but consuming meat naturally provides this beneficial compound, enhancing strength, endurance, and recovery.

The Role of Meat in Muscle Maintenance and Growth

Muscle Protein Synthesis

The high-quality protein in meat stimulates muscle protein synthesis, the process by which the body repairs and builds muscle tissue. This is especially important for maintaining muscle mass as we age, which is crucial for overall health, mobility, and metabolic function.

Preventing Sarcopenia

Sarcopenia, the age-related loss of muscle mass and strength, is a significant concern for older adults. A diet rich in animal protein can help prevent sarcopenia, promoting better physical function, independence, and quality of life in older age.

The Impact of Meat on Metabolic Health

Blood Sugar Regulation

A meat-based diet can help stabilize blood sugar levels by reducing the intake of carbohydrates, which can cause blood sugar spikes and crashes. The consistent intake of protein and fat helps maintain steady energy levels and improves insulin sensitivity, reducing the risk of type 2 diabetes and metabolic syndrome.

Weight Management

The Carnivore diet can support weight loss and weight management through various mechanisms. High-protein diets increase satiety, helping to reduce overall calorie intake. Additionally, the reduction of carbohydrate intake minimizes insulin spikes, promoting fat burning and reducing fat storage.

The Anti-Inflammatory Properties of Meat
Reducing Chronic Inflammation

Chronic inflammation is a root cause of many modern diseases, including heart disease, diabetes, and autoimmune conditions. The Carnivore diet, by eliminating common inflammatory foods such as grains, legumes, and processed sugars, can significantly reduce inflammation. The omega-3 fatty acids found in grass-fed meats and fatty fish also have potent anti-inflammatory effects, supporting overall health and well-being.

Cognitive and Mental Health Benefits

Brain Health and Function

The brain thrives on the nutrients found in meat. Omega-3 fatty acids, B vitamins, and high-quality proteins support cognitive function, mental clarity, and overall brain health. These nutrients help reduce the risk of neurodegenerative diseases such as Alzheimer's and support mood regulation and mental health.

Mood and Mental Well-Being

A diet rich in animal products can positively impact mental health. Adequate intake of omega-3 fatty acids, vitamin B12, and zinc has been linked to reduced symptoms of depression and anxiety. The Carnivore diet's nutrient density provides the brain with the essential building blocks for neurotransmitter production and optimal function.

Practical Benefits of a Meat-Only Diet

Simplified Meal Planning

One of the practical advantages of the Carnivore diet is the simplicity it brings to meal planning. With a focus on meat, fish, eggs, and animal fats, the choices are straightforward, reducing the stress and complexity often associated with meal preparation. This simplicity allows for more consistent adherence to the diet, which is crucial for long-term success.

Cost-Effectiveness

While high-quality animal products can be more expensive than processed foods, the Carnivore diet can be cost-effective in the long run. By eliminating the need for supplements, snacks, and a wide variety of foods, you may find that your overall grocery bill decreases. Investing in nutrient-dense foods also means investing in your long-term health, potentially reducing medical costs associated with poor nutrition.

Addressing Common Concerns

Cholesterol and Heart Health

A common concern about a meat-heavy diet is its impact on cholesterol levels and heart health. However, recent research indicates that the relationship between dietary cholesterol and heart disease is more complex than previously thought. Many individuals on the Carnivore diet experience improvements in lipid profiles, including increased HDL (good) cholesterol and reduced triglycerides, indicating better heart health.

Nutrient Diversity

Some worry that a meat-only diet may lack essential nutrients found in plant foods. However, when consuming a variety of animal products, including organ meats, seafood, and eggs, you can obtain all necessary nutrients. Additionally, the bioavailability of these nutrients in animal products is often higher than in plant foods, meaning your body can absorb and use them more effectively.

The nutritional power of meat is profound and far-reaching. By focusing on high-quality animal products, the Carnivore diet provides all the essential nutrients needed for optimal health. From high-quality protein and healthy fats to vital vitamins and minerals, meat offers a comprehensive nutritional profile that supports muscle maintenance, metabolic health, cognitive function, and overall well-being. Simplifying your diet to focus on these nutrient-dense foods not only enhances physical health but also promotes mental clarity, energy, and long-term vitality. As you continue your journey with the Pure Carnivore lifestyle, remember that the simplicity and nutritional power of meat are your allies in achieving and maintaining optimal health.

Chapter 3

How To Begin Your Carnivore Journey

Practical Steps to Transitioning

Embarking on a carnivore diet journey can be both exciting and daunting. The simplicity of the diet is appealing, but transitioning to a meat-only lifestyle requires preparation and a clear understanding of what to expect. This chapter provides practical steps and advice to help you successfully begin your carnivore journey, from initial planning to navigating potential challenges.

Understanding the Basics

What to Eat

The foundation of the carnivore diet is simple: consume only animal-based foods. **This includes:**

- Meat: Beef, pork, lamb, poultry, and game meats.

- Fish and Seafood: Salmon, tuna, sardines, shrimp, and other seafood.

- Eggs: Chicken, duck, and quail eggs.

- Animal Fats: Butter, ghee, tallow, lard, and suet.

- Organ Meats: Liver, kidneys, heart, and other nutrient-dense organs.

What to Avoid

Equally important is knowing what to avoid. The carnivore diet eliminates all plant-based foods, including:

- Vegetables and Fruits: All types, including leafy greens, root vegetables, and berries.
- Grains: Wheat, rice, oats, and all other grains.
- Legumes: Beans, lentils, peas, and peanuts.
- Nuts and Seeds: Almonds, walnuts, sunflower seeds, and similar foods.
- Processed Foods: Anything with added sugars, artificial additives, or preservatives.

Preparing for the Transition

Educate Yourself

Before you start, it's crucial to educate yourself about the carnivore diet. Read books, listen to podcasts, and follow reputable sources online to understand the diet's principles, benefits, and potential challenges. Knowledge is empowering and will help you make informed decisions throughout your journey.

Plan Your Meals

Meal planning is essential for a successful transition. Start by listing your favorite meats and animal-based foods, and create a weekly meal plan. This will help you stay organized and ensure you have the necessary ingredients on hand. Consider batch cooking and freezing portions for convenience.

Stock Your Kitchen

Stocking your kitchen with high-quality animal products is a critical step. Visit local butchers, farmers' markets, or specialty grocery stores to find the best sources of meat, fish, and eggs. Investing in a freezer can also be beneficial, allowing you to buy in bulk and store your meats for longer periods.

Starting Your Carnivore Journey

Gradual Transition vs. Cold Turkey

Decide whether you want to transition gradually or go cold turkey. A gradual transition involves slowly reducing plant-based foods and increasing your intake of animal products over a few weeks. This approach can help your body adjust and may reduce potential side effects. Going cold turkey, on the other hand, means immediately switching to a meat-only diet. This method may lead to a quicker adaptation but can be more challenging initially.

Hydration and Electrolytes

Staying hydrated is crucial on the carnivore diet. Meat contains less water than many plant foods, so ensure you drink plenty of water throughout the day. Additionally, the diet's diuretic effect can lead to an increased loss of electrolytes, such as sodium, potassium, and magnesium. Consider adding a pinch of salt to your water or consuming electrolyte supplements to maintain balance.

Listen to Your Body

During the initial transition, pay close attention to your body's signals. Some people experience changes in digestion, energy levels, and mood as their bodies adapt to the new diet. Common symptoms include fatigue, headaches, and digestive issues, often referred to as the "carnivore flu." These symptoms typically subside within a few days to weeks as your body adjusts.

Navigating Common Challenges
Social Situations

One of the most significant challenges of the carnivore diet is navigating social situations. Dining out, attending parties, and family gatherings can be tricky. Here are some tips to help you stay on track:

- Research Restaurants: Look for restaurants that offer meat-focused dishes, such as steakhouses or barbecue joints. Call ahead to ask about menu options and accommodations.
- Bring Your Own Food: When attending social events, consider bringing your own food. This ensures you have

something to eat that aligns with your diet and avoids potential temptations.

- Communicate Your Needs: Be open about your dietary choices with friends and family. Explain why you're following the carnivore diet and ask for their support and understanding.

Cravings and Temptations

Cravings for non-carnivore foods are common, especially in the beginning. Here are some strategies to manage them:

- Stay Satiated: Eating enough high-quality protein and fat can help keep you full and reduce cravings. Don't be afraid to eat more meat if you're feeling hungry.
- Find Carnivore-Friendly Alternatives: Satisfy your cravings with carnivore-friendly alternatives. For example, if you're craving something crunchy, try pork rinds. If you miss sweets, consider incorporating fatty cuts of meat that have a natural sweetness.
- Mindset and Motivation: Remind yourself of your reasons for choosing the carnivore diet. Keep a journal of your progress and any positive changes you notice, such as

improved energy levels or better digestion. This can help reinforce your commitment and keep you motivated.

Long-Term Success

Consistency and Routine

Consistency is key to long-term success on the carnivore diet. Establishing a routine can help you stay on track. Plan your meals, set regular eating times, and create habits that support your dietary goals. Over time, these routines will become second nature, making it easier to maintain the diet.

Monitor Your Health

Regularly monitoring your health is essential. Keep track of how you feel physically and mentally, and note any changes in symptoms or energy levels. Consider getting periodic blood tests to monitor your nutrient levels and overall health. Working with a healthcare professional knowledgeable about the carnivore diet can provide additional support and guidance.

Community and Support

Joining a community of like-minded individuals can provide valuable support and motivation. Online forums, social media groups, and local meetups offer opportunities to connect with others who share your commitment to the carnivore diet. Sharing experiences, tips, and recipes can enhance your journey and help you stay motivated.

Transitioning to a carnivore diet is a significant lifestyle change, but with the right preparation and mindset, it can be a rewarding and transformative experience. By understanding the basics, planning your meals, staying hydrated, and listening to your body, you can navigate the challenges and enjoy the benefits of a meat-only diet. Remember that consistency and support are key to long-term success. Embrace the simplicity and nutritional power of the carnivore diet, and begin your journey to amplified health and well-being.

Chapter 4

Essential Nutrients In Animal Foods

Comprehensive Guide to Key Nutrients

Animal foods are a treasure trove of essential nutrients that support a wide range of bodily functions. This chapter delves into the key nutrients found in animal products, explaining their roles, benefits, and how they contribute to overall health. By understanding the nutritional profile of meat, fish, eggs, and other animal foods, you can appreciate the profound impact these foods have on your well-being.

Protein: The Building Block of Life

Complete Amino Acid Profile

Animal foods provide high-quality protein, containing all nine essential amino acids that the body cannot synthesize on its own. These amino acids are critical for:

- Muscle Growth and Repair: Supporting muscle maintenance, recovery, and growth.

- Enzyme Function: Facilitating biochemical reactions necessary for digestion, energy production, and other vital processes.

- Immune System: Producing antibodies that help defend against infections.

Healthy Fats: Essential for Vital Functions

Saturated Fats

Saturated fats in animal foods play essential roles in the body:

- Hormone Production: Essential for the synthesis of hormones like testosterone and estrogen.

- Cell Membrane Integrity: Maintaining the structure and function of cell membranes.

- Brain Health: Providing a critical energy source for the brain.

Monounsaturated Fats

Found in meats and fatty fish, monounsaturated fats offer several health benefits:

- Heart Health: Reducing bad cholesterol levels (LDL) while increasing good cholesterol (HDL).

- Inflammation Reduction: Helping to reduce chronic inflammation linked to various diseases.

Omega-3 and Omega-6 Fatty Acids

These essential fatty acids are crucial for numerous bodily functions:

- Brain Function: Supporting cognitive function and mental health.

- Heart Health: Reducing the risk of heart disease by lowering triglycerides and blood pressure.

- Anti-Inflammatory Properties: Omega-3s, found in fatty fish, are particularly effective in reducing inflammation.

Vitamins: Catalysts for Health

Vitamin B12

Vitamin B12, abundant in animal products, is vital for:

- Red Blood Cell Formation: Preventing anemia and promoting oxygen transport.

- Nervous System Health: Supporting nerve function and preventing neurological disorders.

- DNA Synthesis: Essential for cellular replication and overall growth.

Vitamin A

Animal foods provide preformed vitamin A (retinol), which is crucial for:

- Vision: Maintaining healthy vision and preventing night blindness.
- Immune Function: Enhancing immune response and reducing the risk of infections.
- Skin Health: Promoting skin health and reducing the signs of aging.

Vitamin D

While the body can synthesize vitamin D from sunlight, dietary sources in fatty fish, liver, and egg yolks are also important:

- Bone Health: Regulating calcium and phosphorus levels for strong bones and teeth.
- Immune Function: Boosting the immune system and reducing the risk of chronic diseases.

Vitamin K2

Found in animal products, particularly organ meats and dairy, vitamin K2 is essential for:

- Bone Health: Helping to direct calcium to the bones and teeth, preventing calcification of arteries.

- Cardiovascular Health: Reducing the risk of heart disease by preventing arterial calcification.

Minerals: Building Blocks for Health

Iron

Animal foods, especially red meat, provide heme iron, which is more readily absorbed than non-heme iron from plants:

- Oxygen Transport: Facilitating the transport of oxygen in the blood.

- Energy Production: Supporting metabolic processes and energy levels.

Zinc

Zinc is abundant in meat, shellfish, and dairy, and is essential for:

- Immune Function: Boosting immune response and aiding in wound healing.

- DNA Synthesis: Supporting cell division and growth.

- Reproductive Health: Playing a critical role in hormone production and reproductive health.

Selenium

Found in meat, fish, and eggs, selenium is a powerful antioxidant:

- Thyroid Function: Supporting the production of thyroid hormones.

- Antioxidant Defense: Protecting cells from oxidative stress and reducing the risk of chronic diseases.

Creatine: Enhancing Physical Performance

Creatine, found primarily in red meat and fish, is a key compound for energy production:

- Muscle Energy: Providing quick energy for high-intensity exercise.

- Strength and Endurance: Enhancing physical performance, muscle strength, and recovery.

Cholesterol: Essential for Health

While often misunderstood, cholesterol in animal foods is crucial for:

- Cell Membrane Structure: Maintaining the integrity and fluidity of cell membranes.

- Hormone Production: Serving as a precursor for steroid hormones like cortisol, estrogen, and testosterone.

- Vitamin D Synthesis: Playing a role in the synthesis of

vitamin D in the skin.

 Taurine: Supporting Heart and Brain Health

Taurine, an amino acid found in meat and fish, is important for:

- Cardiovascular Health: Supporting heart function and reducing the risk of heart disease.

- Neurological Function: Aiding in the development and function of the central nervous system.

- Electrolyte Balance: Helping to maintain proper hydration and electrolyte balance.

Glycine: Promoting Joint and Skin Health

Glycine, abundant in collagen-rich animal parts like skin and bones, is vital for:

- Joint Health: Supporting the synthesis of collagen, which is essential for joint health and flexibility.

- Skin Health: Promoting skin elasticity and reducing the signs of aging.

- Detoxification: Aiding in the body's natural detoxification processes.

Carnitine: Enhancing Energy Production

Carnitine, found in red meat, plays a critical role in:

- Fat Metabolism: Transporting fatty acids into mitochondria for energy production.

- Heart Health: Supporting heart function and reducing the risk of heart disease.

- Muscle Function: Enhancing muscle energy and performance.

Animal foods are rich in essential nutrients that support a wide range of bodily functions, from muscle growth and immune function to cognitive health and energy production. By focusing on high-quality meat, fish, eggs, and other animal products, you can ensure that you are providing your body with the nutrients it needs to thrive. Understanding the nutritional power of animal foods reinforces the benefits of the carnivore diet and its potential to amplify your health and well-being. As you continue your journey with the Pure Carnivore lifestyle, remember that these nutrient-dense foods are the foundation of optimal health and vitality.

Chapter 5

Health Transformations

Real-Life Benefits of Simplifying Your Diet

Simplifying your diet by focusing on meat-only nutrition can lead to remarkable health transformations. In this chapter, we'll explore the real-life benefits of adopting a carnivore diet, backed by scientific evidence and personal testimonials. From dramatic weight loss to improved mental clarity, these transformations demonstrate the profound impact that a simplified diet can have on overall health and well-being.

Weight Loss and Body Composition

Fat Loss and Muscle Preservation

One of the most common and immediate benefits of the carnivore diet is weight loss. By eliminating carbohydrates and relying solely on animal-based foods, the body shifts into a state of ketosis, where it burns fat for fuel instead of glucose. This metabolic switch promotes significant fat loss while preserving lean muscle mass. Numerous individuals have reported:

- Rapid Weight Loss: Many experience a significant drop in weight within the first few weeks of adopting the carnivore diet.

- Improved Body Composition: Reduced body fat percentage and increased muscle definition.

Testimonial: Sarah's Transformation

Sarah struggled with her weight for years, trying various diets with limited success. After switching to a carnivore diet, she lost 30 pounds in three months. "Not only did I shed the weight, but I also felt stronger and more energetic than ever before," she says. "My body composition improved dramatically."

Enhanced Mental Clarity and Cognitive Function

Mental Focus and Sharpness

Another profound benefit of the carnivore diet is enhanced mental clarity. Many people report improved focus, memory, and overall cognitive function. This cognitive boost is likely due to the stabilization of blood sugar levels and the anti-inflammatory effects of a meat-based diet. Benefits include:

- Steady Energy Levels: Eliminating carbohydrates prevents blood sugar spikes and crashes, leading to sustained mental energy.
- Reduced Brain Fog: Many find that brain fog lifts, making it easier to concentrate and think clearly.

Testimonial: John's Cognitive Revival

John, a software engineer, found his productivity plummeting due to constant brain fog and fatigue. "Switching to the carnivore diet was a game-changer," he shares. "My mind feels sharper, and I can work for hours without feeling drained."

Improved Digestion and Gut Health

Alleviating Digestive Issues

Digestive issues such as bloating, gas, and irritable bowel syndrome (IBS) can be debilitating. The carnivore diet, with its elimination of plant fibers and antinutrients, often leads to significant improvements in gut health. Individuals have reported:

- Reduced Bloating: The absence of fermentable fibers and sugars reduces gas production and bloating.
- Relief from IBS Symptoms: Many find that symptoms of IBS, such as cramping and irregular bowel movements, improve or disappear entirely.

Testimonial: Emily's Digestive Relief

Emily suffered from chronic bloating and IBS for years. "Within weeks of starting the carnivore diet, my digestive issues were gone," she says. "I feel lighter and more comfortable after meals."

Enhanced Physical Performance
Strength, Endurance, and Recovery

Athletes and fitness enthusiasts often notice significant improvements in their physical performance on a carnivore diet. The high protein intake supports muscle growth and repair, while the stable energy supply from fats enhances endurance. Benefits include:
- Increased Strength: Higher protein intake aids in muscle building and strength gains.

- Improved Endurance: Steady energy from fat metabolism supports prolonged physical activity.

- Faster Recovery: Reduced inflammation and adequate nutrient intake promote quicker recovery from workouts.

Testimonial: Mike's Athletic Edge

Mike, a competitive powerlifter, struggled with recovery and performance plateaus. "Since switching to a carnivore diet, my lifts have gone up, and I recover faster between workouts," he reports. "I feel stronger and more resilient."

Skin Health and Anti-Aging

Radiant Skin and Reduced Signs of Aging

A meat-based diet can also have remarkable effects on skin health. The nutrient-dense nature of animal foods, rich in vitamins A, D, E, and K2, supports skin health and reduces signs of aging. Benefits include:

- Clearer Skin: Many experience fewer breakouts and improved skin clarity.

- Youthful Appearance: Increased collagen intake from animal foods promotes skin elasticity and reduces wrinkles.

Testimonial: Lisa's Skin Transformation

Lisa, who battled with acne and premature aging signs, noticed dramatic improvements after adopting a carnivore diet. "My skin is clearer, and I look younger," she says. "It's like I found the fountain of youth in my diet."

Enhanced Immune Function

Strengthening the Body's Defenses

A diet rich in high-quality animal foods can bolster the immune system. Essential nutrients like zinc, selenium, and vitamin A play critical roles in immune function. Individuals on a carnivore diet often report:

- Fewer Illnesses: Enhanced resistance to common colds and infections.

- Faster Recovery: Quicker recovery times from illnesses and injuries.

Testimonial: Dave's Immune Boost

Dave, who frequently fell ill, found his health improving on a carnivore diet. "I used to catch colds all the time, but now I rarely get sick," he shares. "My immune system feels stronger than ever."

Hormonal Balance and Vitality

Regulating Hormones Naturally

The carnivore diet can help balance hormones, leading to improved energy levels, mood, and overall vitality. Key benefits include:

- Stabilized Blood Sugar: Reducing carbohydrate intake helps regulate insulin levels.

- Hormonal Harmony: Adequate intake of cholesterol and saturated fats supports hormone production.

Testimonial: Maria's Hormonal Harmony

Maria, who struggled with hormonal imbalances and mood swings, found relief with the carnivore diet. "My energy levels are stable, and my mood has improved," she says. "I feel balanced and vibrant."

The health transformations associated with the carnivore diet are profound and far-reaching. From weight loss and enhanced mental clarity to improved digestion and physical performance, simplifying your diet by focusing on nutrient-dense animal foods can lead to remarkable benefits. These real-life success stories highlight the potential of the carnivore diet to amplify health and well-being. As you continue your journey, embrace the simplicity and power of this dietary approach, and witness your own health transformation unfold.

Chapter 6

Mental Clarity And Focus

How a Simplified Diet Enhances Cognitive Function

Mental clarity and focus are often elusive in today's fast-paced, high-stress world. However, many individuals report significant improvements in their cognitive function upon adopting a carnivore diet. This chapter explores how simplifying your diet to include only animal-based foods can lead to enhanced mental performance, better focus, and overall cognitive well-being. We'll delve into the science behind these benefits and share real-life experiences from those who have experienced a mental transformation.

Stabilizing Blood Sugar Levels

The Role of Carbohydrates in Cognitive Function

Carbohydrates, particularly refined sugars, can cause rapid spikes and drops in blood sugar levels. These fluctuations can lead to periods of hyperactivity followed by crashes, which negatively affect cognitive function. Symptoms include:

- Brain Fog: Difficulty concentrating and thinking clearly.

- Energy Slumps: Fatigue and lethargy during the day.

By eliminating carbohydrates and relying on a diet rich in animal fats and proteins, you stabilize blood sugar levels, leading to sustained energy and improved mental clarity.

Scientific Insight

Research has shown that a diet low in carbohydrates and high in fats can lead to better cognitive function by providing a steady supply of energy to the brain. The brain primarily relies on glucose for energy, but it can efficiently use ketones, derived from fat, when glucose is not readily available.

Enhancing Neurotransmitter Function

The Impact of Nutrients on Brain Health

Animal foods are rich in nutrients that support the production and function of neurotransmitters, the chemicals that transmit signals in the brain. Key nutrients include:

- Omega-3 Fatty Acids: Found in fatty fish and grass-fed meats, these fats are essential for brain health and function. They support the structure of brain cells and are involved in the production of neurotransmitters like serotonin and dopamine.

- Vitamin B12: Crucial for the maintenance of myelin, the protective sheath around nerve fibers, and for overall brain function. Deficiency in B12 can lead to cognitive impairments and mood disorders.

Testimonial: Mark's Cognitive Awakening

Mark, a college professor, struggled with focus and memory retention. After adopting the carnivore diet, he noticed a dramatic improvement. "My ability to concentrate and retain information has skyrocketed," he says. "I feel sharper and more mentally agile than I have in years."

Reducing Inflammation

The Anti-Inflammatory Benefits of the Carnivore Diet

Chronic inflammation is linked to numerous cognitive disorders, including Alzheimer's disease and depression. The carnivore diet, devoid of inflammatory plant compounds and rich in anti-inflammatory nutrients, can help reduce brain inflammation, leading to improved cognitive function.

Scientific Insight

Studies have shown that diets high in omega-3 fatty acids and low in processed foods can reduce markers of inflammation in the body. This reduction in inflammation is associated with better cognitive performance and a lower risk of neurodegenerative diseases.

Improving Gut Health

The Gut-Brain Connection

The gut-brain axis is a complex communication network linking the gastrointestinal tract and the brain. Gut health significantly impacts cognitive function and mood. The carnivore diet can improve gut health by eliminating plant fibers and antinutrients that may cause digestive issues and inflammation.

Testimonial: Jane's Gut-Brain Revival

Jane, who suffered from irritable bowel syndrome (IBS) and brain fog, experienced remarkable improvements after switching to a carnivore diet. "My digestive issues vanished, and my mind became clearer," she shares. "It's incredible how closely linked our gut and brain are."

Boosting Energy Levels

The Role of Ketosis in Cognitive Performance

The carnivore diet often induces a state of ketosis, where the body burns fat for fuel instead of carbohydrates. Ketones, the byproducts of fat metabolism, are a more efficient and stable energy source for the brain.

Scientific Insight

Research suggests that ketones can enhance mitochondrial function and reduce oxidative stress in the brain, leading to improved cognitive performance. People on ketogenic diets often report better mental clarity, focus, and overall brain function.

Enhancing Mental Resilience

The Psychological Benefits of a Simplified Diet

Adopting a carnivore diet simplifies food choices, reducing the mental burden of deciding what to eat and potentially reducing anxiety related to food choices and dietary restrictions. This simplification can lead to better mental resilience and a more focused mind.

Testimonial: David's Mental Calm

David, who felt overwhelmed by the complexity of various diets, found peace and mental clarity in the simplicity of the carnivore diet. "Not having to worry about what to eat and knowing that I'm nourishing my body properly has lifted a huge weight off my shoulders," he says. "I can focus on more important things."

Cognitive Benefits Across All Ages

From Youth to Seniors

The cognitive benefits of the carnivore diet are not limited to any specific age group. From improved focus in children and adolescents to enhanced memory and reduced cognitive decline in older adults, the benefits are wide-reaching.

Testimonial: Emily's Academic Edge

Emily, a high school student, struggled with concentration and energy levels during her studies. After transitioning to a carnivore diet, she noticed a significant improvement. "My grades improved, and I felt more focused and energized throughout the day," she shares. "It's like a fog has lifted."

Testimonial: Richard's Senior Clarity

Richard, in his 70s, experienced memory lapses and cognitive decline. After adopting a carnivore diet, he noticed improved mental clarity and better recall. "I feel like my mind is sharper, and I'm more present in my daily activities," he says. "It's been a remarkable change."

Simplifying your diet to focus on nutrient-dense animal foods can lead to significant improvements in mental clarity, focus, and overall cognitive function. The benefits of stabilizing blood sugar levels, reducing inflammation, enhancing neurotransmitter function, and improving gut health all contribute to a sharper, more focused mind. These real-life testimonials and scientific insights highlight the potential of the carnivore diet to transform cognitive health and enhance mental performance across all ages. Embrace the simplicity and power of this dietary approach, and experience the mental clarity and focus that come with a pure carnivore lifestyle.

Chapter 7

Improving Energy Levels

Sustained Energy with the Carnivore Diet

Energy levels play a crucial role in how we navigate our daily lives, from work and exercise to personal activities and mental tasks. A diet that provides consistent and sustained energy can significantly enhance productivity, physical performance, and overall well-being. The carnivore diet, with its unique nutritional profile, offers a powerful way to achieve these goals. This chapter explores how a meat-only diet can improve energy levels, stabilize blood sugar, and promote overall vitality.

The Problem with Carbohydrates

Blood Sugar Spikes and Crashes

Many diets rely heavily on carbohydrates, which can cause significant fluctuations in blood sugar levels. When you consume carbs, your body converts them into glucose, which spikes your blood sugar. This spike triggers the release of insulin to help cells absorb the glucose, often leading to a rapid drop in blood sugar levels, known as a crash. These crashes can cause:

- Fatigue: Sudden drops in energy levels.

- Irritability: Mood swings and irritability due to unstable blood sugar.

- Hunger: Increased hunger and cravings for more carbohydrates.

The Ketogenic Advantage

Steady Energy from Fat Metabolism

The carnivore diet often induces a state of ketosis, where the body burns fat for fuel instead of carbohydrates. In ketosis, the liver converts fats into ketones, which serve as a stable and efficient energy source. The benefits of ketosis include:

- Consistent Energy Levels: Without the spikes and crashes associated with carbohydrate consumption, energy levels remain steady throughout the day.

- Reduced Hunger: Ketones help regulate appetite, leading to reduced hunger and cravings.

Scientific Insight

Studies have shown that ketogenic diets can lead to improved energy levels and reduced feelings of fatigue. This is particularly beneficial for individuals who engage in prolonged physical activities or mentally demanding tasks.

The Role of Protein

Sustained Energy from High-Quality Protein

Meat is a rich source of high-quality protein, which is essential for maintaining muscle mass, repairing tissues, and supporting various bodily functions. Protein provides a more sustained energy release compared to carbohydrates, helping to keep you feeling fuller for longer and providing a steady supply of amino acids to your muscles and organs.

Testimonial: Laura's Protein Power

Laura, a marathon runner, found her energy levels fluctuating on a high-carb diet. After switching to a carnivore diet, she noticed a significant improvement. "My energy is much more consistent, and I no longer experience the mid-run crashes," she says. "Protein has become my secret weapon for endurance."

Essential Nutrients in Meat

Vitamins and Minerals for Energy Production

Animal foods are rich in essential vitamins and minerals that play critical roles in energy production and overall health. **Key nutrients include:**

- Iron: Essential for oxygen transport in the blood, iron helps prevent fatigue and supports physical performance.

- Vitamin B12: Crucial for red blood cell formation and neurological function, B12 deficiencies can lead to fatigue and weakness.

- Zinc and Magnesium: Important for enzyme function and energy metabolism, these minerals support muscle function and overall vitality.

Scientific Insight

Research indicates that deficiencies in essential nutrients like iron and B12 are common in non-meat diets and can lead to chronic fatigue and reduced energy levels. Consuming a nutrient-dense carnivore diet can help prevent these deficiencies and support sustained energy.

Enhancing Mitochondrial Function

The Powerhouses of the Cell

Mitochondria, often referred to as the powerhouses of the cell, play a vital role in energy production. A diet rich in healthy fats and proteins can support mitochondrial function, leading to improved energy production and reduced oxidative stress.

Scientific Insight

Studies have shown that ketogenic diets can enhance mitochondrial function and reduce oxidative stress, leading to improved energy production and endurance.

The Anti-Inflammatory Effects

Reducing Inflammation for Better Energy

Chronic inflammation can drain your energy and contribute to feelings of fatigue and lethargy. The carnivore diet, which eliminates inflammatory plant compounds and is rich in anti-inflammatory nutrients, can help reduce overall inflammation in the body.

Testimonial: Paul's Energy Revival

Paul, who suffered from chronic fatigue and joint pain, found significant relief after adopting a carnivore diet. "My inflammation levels have dropped, and I feel more energized than I have in years," he shares. "I wake up feeling refreshed and ready to tackle the day."

Adapting to the Carnivore Diet

The Transition Period

While the carnivore diet can lead to sustained energy levels, there is often an adaptation period as your body adjusts to burning fat for fuel. During this period, some individuals may experience temporary fatigue or what is commonly referred to as the "keto flu." This transition typically includes symptoms like:

- Fatigue: Temporary energy dips as the body adapts.

- Headaches: Due to changes in electrolyte levels.

- Irritability: As the body adjusts to a new fuel source.

Tips for a Smooth Transition

To minimize these effects, it's essential to stay hydrated, consume adequate electrolytes (sodium, potassium, and magnesium), and ensure you're eating enough fat and protein to meet your energy needs.

Practical Tips for Sustained Energy

Making the Most of Your Carnivore Diet

To maximize the energy benefits of the carnivore diet, consider the following practical tips:

- Stay Hydrated: Drink plenty of water to support energy levels and overall health.

- Consume Adequate Fat: Ensure you're getting enough healthy fats from sources like fatty cuts of meat, butter, and animal-based oils to maintain ketosis and energy levels.

- Eat Organ Meats: Incorporate nutrient-dense organ meats like liver and kidney, which are rich in vitamins and minerals essential for energy production.

- Listen to Your Body: Pay attention to hunger cues and eat when you're hungry. The carnivore diet naturally regulates appetite, so trust your body's signals.

Testimonial: Sarah's Sustained Energy

Sarah, a busy mother of three, struggled with energy crashes and constant fatigue. After switching to a carnivore diet, she noticed a remarkable difference. "I have steady energy throughout the day, and I no longer feel the need for afternoon naps," she says. "It's been a game-changer for managing my busy lifestyle."

The carnivore diet offers a powerful way to achieve sustained energy levels and enhance overall vitality. By stabilizing blood sugar, providing high-quality protein, and supplying essential nutrients, a meat-only diet can help you maintain consistent energy throughout the day. As you embrace the carnivore lifestyle, you'll likely experience a significant boost in energy, allowing you to perform at your best in all aspects of life. Embrace the simplicity and power of the carnivore diet and enjoy the sustained energy and vitality that come with it.

Chapter 8

Digestive Health

Healing Your Gut with Animal-Based Nutrition

Digestive health is the cornerstone of overall well-being. A properly functioning digestive system ensures efficient nutrient absorption, supports immune function, and contributes to mental health. Many individuals struggle with digestive issues such as bloating, gas, constipation, and inflammatory bowel diseases. This chapter explores how a carnivore diet can heal your gut, reduce inflammation, and promote optimal digestive health through animal-based nutrition.

The Problem with Plant-Based Foods

Fiber and Antinutrients

Many modern diets emphasize plant-based foods, which are high in fiber and antinutrients. While fiber is often touted for its digestive benefits, it can actually cause issues for many people. Antinutrients, on the other hand, can interfere with nutrient absorption and contribute to gut irritation.

- Fiber: Although fiber is believed to aid digestion, it can cause bloating, gas, and constipation for some individuals. Excessive fiber intake can also irritate the gut lining, leading to inflammation.

- Antinutrients: Compounds like lectins, oxalates, and phytates, found in plant foods, can hinder nutrient absorption and contribute to digestive discomfort.

Scientific Insight

Research suggests that some individuals with irritable bowel syndrome (IBS) or other gut issues may benefit from reducing or eliminating fiber from their diet. Additionally, antinutrients in plants can exacerbate digestive problems by binding to minerals and preventing their absorption.

The Gut-Healing Power of Meat

Low Residue and Easy Digestion

Meat is inherently low in fiber and antinutrients, making it easier to digest and less likely to irritate the gut. A carnivore diet focuses on nutrient-dense animal foods that are gentle on the digestive system.

- Low Residue: Meat leaves minimal residue in the digestive tract, reducing the likelihood of bloating and constipation.
- Easy Digestion: Animal proteins and fats are efficiently broken down and absorbed, minimizing digestive discomfort.

Testimonial: Amy's Gut Transformation

Amy, who suffered from chronic bloating and constipation, found relief after transitioning to a carnivore diet. "I no longer feel bloated after meals, and my digestion has improved dramatically," she shares. "It's like my gut has finally found peace."

Reducing Inflammation

The Anti-Inflammatory Benefits of Animal Foods

Chronic inflammation in the gut can lead to conditions like IBS, Crohn's disease, and ulcerative colitis. The carnivore diet, devoid of inflammatory plant compounds, helps reduce gut inflammation and promotes healing.

Scientific Insight

Studies have shown that diets high in omega-3 fatty acids and low in inflammatory compounds can reduce gut inflammation and improve symptoms of inflammatory bowel diseases. Animal foods, particularly fatty fish and grass-fed meats, are rich sources of these beneficial fats.

Balancing Gut Microbiota
The Role of Animal-Based Nutrition

The gut microbiota, a complex community of microorganisms, plays a crucial role in digestive health. A balanced gut microbiota supports nutrient absorption, immune function, and overall gut health. The carnivore diet can help rebalance the gut microbiota by reducing the intake of fermentable fibers that feed harmful bacteria.

Testimonial: John's Microbiome Miracle

John, who struggled with dysbiosis and frequent digestive issues, noticed significant improvements after adopting a carnivore diet. "My gut health has improved, and I no longer suffer from constant discomfort," he says. "My microbiome feels more balanced and stable."

Enhancing Nutrient Absorption

Maximizing Bioavailability

One of the key benefits of a carnivore diet is the bioavailability of nutrients in animal foods. Nutrients from meat are more easily absorbed and utilized by the body compared to plant-based sources, which can be hindered by antinutrients.

- Heme Iron: Found in red meat, heme iron is more readily absorbed than non-heme iron from plant sources.
- Vitamin B12: Abundant in animal foods, vitamin B12 is essential for digestive health and is not found in plant foods.
- Amino Acids: Animal proteins provide a complete profile of essential amino acids necessary for gut repair and overall health.

Scientific Insight

Research indicates that individuals following a meat-based diet often have better iron and B12 status, which are critical for maintaining energy levels and preventing anemia. These nutrients are crucial for gut health and overall well-being.

Healing Leaky Gut

Sealing the Gut Lining

Leaky gut syndrome, characterized by increased intestinal permeability, allows toxins and undigested food particles to enter the bloodstream, leading to inflammation and various health issues. The carnivore diet can help heal and seal the gut lining, reducing symptoms of leaky gut.

Testimonial: Rachel's Leaky Gut Recovery

Rachel, who experienced symptoms of leaky gut, found relief on the carnivore diet. "My digestive issues have significantly improved, and I feel more energetic and less inflamed," she shares. "The carnivore diet has been a game-changer for my gut health."

Practical Tips for Optimizing Digestive Health

Implementing the Carnivore Diet

To maximize the gut-healing benefits of the carnivore diet, consider the following practical tips:

- Start Slowly: Transition gradually to allow your digestive system to adapt.

- Focus on Quality: Choose high-quality, grass-fed meats and organ meats for maximum nutrient density.

- Stay Hydrated: Drink plenty of water to support digestion and overall health.

- Listen to Your Body: Pay attention to how your body responds and adjust your diet accordingly.

Testimonial: Michael's Digestive Renewal

Michael, who dealt with severe digestive discomfort, experienced a remarkable transformation after switching to a carnivore diet. "I no longer suffer from bloating or pain, and my overall digestion has improved," he says. "It's amazing how a simple dietary change can have such a profound impact."

The carnivore diet offers a powerful approach to healing the gut and improving digestive health. By eliminating problematic plant foods and focusing on nutrient-dense animal foods, you can reduce inflammation, enhance nutrient absorption, and support a balanced gut microbiota.

As you embrace the carnivore lifestyle, you'll likely experience significant improvements in your digestive health, leading to better overall well-being. Embrace the simplicity and power of animal-based nutrition, and enjoy the benefits of a healthy, thriving gut.

Chapter 9

Strengthening Immunity

Boosting Your Immune System Naturally

A robust immune system is essential for protecting the body against infections, diseases, and other health threats. While many factors influence immune health, diet plays a critical role. The carnivore diet, rich in essential nutrients and devoid of inflammatory foods, can significantly boost your immune system naturally. This chapter delves into how animal-based nutrition can enhance immunity, reduce inflammation, and promote overall health.

The Immune System: An Overview

Understanding Immune Function

The immune system is a complex network of cells, tissues, and organs that work together to defend the body against harmful invaders. It consists of two main components:

- Innate Immunity: The body's first line of defense, providing immediate, non-specific protection against pathogens.

- Adaptive Immunity: A more specialized response that develops over time, providing long-term immunity and memory against specific pathogens.

Scientific Insight

Research has shown that a well-nourished immune system can respond more effectively to infections and reduce the risk of chronic diseases. Nutrient deficiencies, on the other hand, can impair immune function and increase susceptibility to illness.

The Role of Animal-Based Nutrition

Essential Nutrients for Immune Health

Animal foods are rich in essential nutrients that support immune function. Key nutrients include:

- Protein: Necessary for the production of immune cells and antibodies.

- Vitamin A: Supports the integrity of mucosal surfaces and enhances the function of white blood cells.

- Vitamin D: Modulates the immune response and reduces inflammation.

- Zinc: Crucial for the development and function of immune cells.

- Omega-3 Fatty Acids: Anti-inflammatory properties that support immune health.

Scientific Insight

Studies indicate that diets rich in these nutrients can enhance immune function, reduce inflammation, and improve overall health outcomes. Animal-based foods provide these nutrients in highly bioavailable forms, ensuring efficient absorption and utilization by the body.

Protein: The Building Block of Immunity

Supporting Immune Cell Production

Protein is essential for the growth, maintenance, and repair of tissues, including those involved in the immune response. Amino acids, the building blocks of protein, are required for the production of immune cells, antibodies, and cytokines.

Testimonial: Kevin's Immune Boost

Kevin, who frequently experienced colds and infections, noticed a significant improvement in his immune health after adopting a carnivore diet. "I feel stronger and more resilient," he says. "I rarely get sick, and my overall health has improved."

Vitamin A: Enhancing Mucosal Immunity

Protecting the Body's Barriers

Vitamin A plays a crucial role in maintaining the integrity of mucosal surfaces, such as those in the respiratory and digestive tracts. These surfaces act as physical barriers to pathogens. Vitamin A also enhances the function of white blood cells, which are essential for the immune response.

Scientific Insight

Research shows that adequate vitamin A levels are associated with reduced risk of infections, particularly in the respiratory and gastrointestinal tracts. Liver, a nutrient-dense organ meat, is an excellent source of bioavailable vitamin A.

Vitamin D: Modulating Immune Response

The Sunshine Vitamin's Role

Vitamin D is known for its role in bone health, but it also plays a critical role in immune function. It modulates the immune response, enhancing the pathogen-fighting effects of monocytes and macrophages while reducing inflammation.

Testimonial: Lisa's Vitamin D Discovery

Lisa, who suffered from frequent infections, found relief after incorporating more vitamin D-rich foods into her diet. "Since adding more fatty fish and liver to my meals, I feel healthier and less prone to getting sick," she shares.

Zinc: A Critical Mineral for Immunity

Supporting Immune Cell Function

Zinc is essential for the development and function of immune cells, including T cells and natural killer cells. It also acts as an antioxidant, protecting immune cells from oxidative stress.

Scientific Insight

Studies indicate that zinc supplementation can reduce the duration and severity of common colds and other infections. Red meat, shellfish, and organ meats are excellent sources of bioavailable zinc.

Omega-3 Fatty Acids: Reducing Inflammation

Anti-Inflammatory Benefits

Omega-3 fatty acids, found in fatty fish and grass-fed meats, have potent anti-inflammatory properties. Chronic inflammation can impair immune function, making it harder for the body to fight off infections and diseases.

Testimonial: Sarah's Inflammation Relief

Sarah, who dealt with chronic inflammation and frequent illnesses, noticed significant improvements after increasing her intake of omega-3-rich foods. "My inflammation has reduced, and I feel more resilient against infections," she says. "The carnivore diet has made a huge difference."

Gut Health and Immunity

The Gut-Immune Connection

A healthy gut is essential for a strong immune system. The gut-associated lymphoid tissue (GALT) plays a crucial role in immune function, housing a significant portion of the body's immune cells. A carnivore diet can support gut health by reducing inflammation, promoting a balanced microbiome, and providing essential nutrients.

Scientific Insight

Research has shown that a healthy gut microbiome supports immune function and reduces the risk of autoimmune and inflammatory diseases. The carnivore diet, by promoting gut health, can enhance overall immune resilience.

Practical Tips for Boosting Immunity on a Carnivore Diet

Implementing Immune-Boosting Strategies

To maximize the immune-boosting benefits of the carnivore diet, consider the following practical tips:

- Focus on Nutrient-Dense Foods: Include a variety of meats, organ meats, and fatty fish to ensure a wide range of essential nutrients.

- Stay Hydrated: Adequate hydration is crucial for maintaining overall health and supporting immune function.

- Get Sunlight: Spend time outdoors to boost your vitamin D levels naturally.

- Manage Stress: Chronic stress can weaken the immune system, so practice stress-reducing techniques such as mindfulness, exercise, and adequate sleep.

- Stay Active: Regular physical activity supports immune health and overall well-being.

Testimonial: Mark's Immune Transformation

Mark, who had a weakened immune system due to chronic stress and poor diet, experienced a significant improvement after adopting a carnivore diet and implementing these strategies. "I feel stronger, healthier, and more resilient," he says. "My immune system is finally functioning at its best."

The carnivore diet offers a powerful way to naturally boost your immune system and enhance overall health. By providing essential nutrients, reducing inflammation, and supporting gut health, a meat-based diet can help you achieve a robust and resilient immune system. As you embrace the carnivore lifestyle, you'll likely experience fewer illnesses, faster recovery times, and better overall vitality. Trust in the power of animal-based nutrition to support your immune health and enjoy the benefits of a strong, healthy body.

Chapter 10

Carnivore Meal Planning

Keeping It Simple in the Kitchen

Embarking on a carnivore diet means rethinking your approach to meal planning and preparation. The beauty of this diet lies in its simplicity—focusing on nutrient-dense animal foods allows you to streamline your kitchen efforts and still reap tremendous health benefits. In this chapter, we'll explore practical tips and strategies for effective carnivore meal planning, ensuring you can maintain a balanced and satisfying diet without complexity.

The Simplicity of Carnivore Eating

Why Simplicity Matters

One of the greatest advantages of the carnivore diet is its straightforward nature. By eliminating the need for elaborate recipes and long ingredient lists, you can reduce decision fatigue, save time, and focus on enjoying your meals.

Scientific Insight

Studies show that dietary simplicity can lead to greater adherence to a diet, which is crucial for long-term success. Simplifying meal planning can reduce stress and make healthy eating more sustainable.

Stocking Your Kitchen

Essential Staples

A well-stocked kitchen is key to staying on track with the carnivore diet. Here are some staples to keep on hand:

- Meats: Beef, pork, lamb, chicken, turkey
- Seafood: Salmon, sardines, mackerel, shrimp
- Organ Meats: Liver, heart, kidneys
- Eggs: Pasture-raised or organic
- Fats: Butter, ghee, tallow, lard
- Bone Broth: Homemade or high-quality store-bought

Testimonial: Jane's Efficient Kitchen

Jane, a busy professional, found that stocking up on these essentials made her meal planning much more manageable.

"Having a variety of meats and fats readily available means I can quickly prepare nutritious meals without stress," she says.

Meal Planning Basics

Creating a Weekly Plan

Planning your meals for the week can help ensure variety and balance, and reduce the temptation to stray from your diet. Here's how to create a simple weekly meal plan:

1. Choose Your Proteins: Select a variety of meats and seafood to keep your meals interesting and nutritionally diverse.

2. Incorporate Organ Meats: Plan to include organ meats at least a couple of times a week for their nutrient density.

3. Schedule Cooking Days: Dedicate a couple of days a week to batch-cooking and meal prep.

Example Meal Plan:

- Monday: Ribeye steak, shrimp, and butter

- Tuesday: Ground beef patties, chicken liver, and ghee

- Wednesday: Lamb chops, sardines, and tallow

- Thursday: Pork belly, salmon, and bone broth

- Friday: Beef short ribs, turkey breast, and lard

- Saturday: Chicken thighs, beef heart, and butter

- Sunday: Bison steak, cod, and ghee

Simplifying Cooking Methods

Easy Cooking Techniques

Keeping cooking methods simple not only saves time but also preserves the nutritional integrity of your food. Here are some easy techniques:

- Grilling: Perfect for steaks, chops, and seafood.
- Baking: Ideal for larger cuts of meat and whole chickens.
- Pan-Frying: Quick and efficient for burgers, liver, and eggs.
- Slow Cooking: Great for tougher cuts like brisket and pork shoulder.
- Broiling: Excellent for achieving a crispy exterior on steaks and fish.

Testimonial: Tom's Cooking Routine

Tom, a carnivore diet enthusiast, streamlined his cooking methods to save time and effort. "I focus on grilling and baking most of my meals. It's quick, easy, and the food tastes fantastic," he shares.

Batch Cooking and Meal Prep
Saving Time and Effort

Batch cooking is a game-changer for busy individuals. By preparing multiple meals at once, you can ensure you have nutritious food ready to go throughout the week.

- Cook in Batches: Prepare large quantities of meats and store them in the refrigerator or freezer.
- Portion Out Meals: Divide your cooked meats into individual portions for easy reheating.
- Use Leftovers: Incorporate leftover meats into different meals to add variety without extra effort.

Testimonial: Emma's Batch Cooking Success

Emma, who juggles a demanding job and family life, found that batch cooking made sticking to the carnivore diet much easier. "I cook a lot on Sundays, and it sets me up for the entire week. It's a lifesaver," she says.

Eating Out on a Carnivore Diet

Navigating Restaurants

While eating out can be challenging on a carnivore diet, it's entirely possible with a few strategies:

- Choose the Right Restaurants: Opt for steakhouses, barbecue joints, and seafood restaurants that offer meat-centric menus.
- Simple Orders: Order plain, grilled, or roasted meats and ask for butter or olive oil instead of sauces.
- Communicate Your Needs: Don't hesitate to ask the server to modify dishes to fit your dietary preferences.

Testimonial: Alex's Dining Out Tips

Alex, who travels frequently for work, developed effective strategies for dining out. "I always research restaurants ahead of time and communicate my needs clearly. It's helped me stay on track even when I'm on the road," he explains.

Managing Cravings and Snacking

Staying Satisfied

The high protein and fat content of the carnivore diet can help manage hunger and reduce cravings. However, if you do feel the need to snack, consider these options:

- Beef Jerky: Opt for homemade or clean-ingredient store-bought options.
- Hard-Boiled Eggs: Easy to prepare and portable.
- Pork Rinds: A crunchy, satisfying snack.
- Cold Cuts: Choose nitrate-free options for a quick protein boost.

Testimonial: Rachel's Snacking Strategy

Rachel, who often experienced afternoon cravings, found that incorporating high-protein snacks helped her stay satisfied. "Beef jerky and hard-boiled eggs have become my go-to snacks. They're filling and keep me on track," she says.

Budget-Friendly Carnivore Eating

Cost-Effective Strategies

Eating a carnivore diet doesn't have to break the bank. Here are some tips for budget-friendly carnivore eating:

- Buy in Bulk: Purchase larger cuts of meat or buy meat in bulk from local farmers or butchers.
- Utilize Cheaper Cuts: Opt for less expensive cuts like ground beef, chuck roast, and pork shoulder.
- Embrace Organ Meats: These nutrient-dense options are often more affordable.
- Shop Sales: Keep an eye out for sales and stock up when prices are lower.

Testimonial: Jason's Budget Tips

Jason, who was concerned about the cost of a carnivore diet, discovered that with careful planning, it was manageable. "Buying in bulk and choosing cheaper cuts has made a big difference. I eat well without overspending," he shares.

Seasonal and Local Eating

Supporting Sustainable Practices

Eating seasonally and locally not only supports sustainable practices but can also enhance the freshness and quality of your food. Here's how to incorporate this into your carnivore diet:

- Local Farmers: Purchase meat from local farmers' markets or farm co-ops.

- Seasonal Seafood: Choose seafood that is in season for optimal freshness.

- Hunting and Fishing: If possible, consider hunting or fishing for a sustainable source of meat.

Testimonial: Sarah's Local Approach

Sarah, who values sustainability, embraced local and seasonal eating. "I buy most of my meat from local farmers, and it's not only fresher but also supports the local economy," she says.

The carnivore diet's simplicity extends to the kitchen, where meal planning and preparation can be straightforward and stress-free. By focusing on essential staples, utilizing simple cooking methods, and planning ahead, you can enjoy a balanced and satisfying diet without complexity. Whether you're cooking at home, dining out, or managing cravings, the strategies outlined in this chapter will help you stay on track and enjoy the benefits of carnivore eating. Embrace the simplicity and efficiency of the carnivore diet, and discover how easy and enjoyable healthy eating can be.

Chapter 11

Social Dynamics and the Carnivore Diet

Navigating Social Situations

Adopting a carnivore diet can be transformative for your health, but it also comes with its unique social challenges. From dining out with friends to family gatherings and office parties, navigating social situations while sticking to your dietary principles requires strategy and confidence. This chapter explores practical tips and advice for maintaining your carnivore lifestyle in a variety of social contexts, ensuring you can enjoy your social life without compromising your dietary goals.

The Social Challenge

Understanding the Social Dynamics

Food is deeply embedded in social interactions, and dietary choices often come under scrutiny. The carnivore diet, with its emphasis on meat and exclusion of plant-based foods, can be particularly polarizing.

Scientific Insight

Studies have shown that social support and acceptance play a significant role in dietary adherence and long-term success. Understanding and preparing for social dynamics can help you stay committed to your diet.

Educating Friends and Family

Communicating Your Choice

When adopting the carnivore diet, it's essential to communicate your reasons and goals clearly to friends and family. Providing them with information can help them understand and support your decision.

Tips for Communication:

1. Be Honest and Open: Explain why you've chosen the carnivore diet and the benefits you've experienced.

2. Provide Resources: Share articles, books, or documentaries that explain the diet's principles.

3. Invite Curiosity: Encourage questions and be prepared to discuss your experiences positively.

Testimonial: Laura's Approach

Laura found that educating her family about her dietary choices helped gain their support. "I took the time to explain why I'm doing this and how it's helped me. Now, they're more understanding and even curious about trying it themselves," she says.

Dining Out with Friends

Strategies for Eating Out

Eating out can be one of the biggest challenges on a carnivore diet, but with some planning, it's entirely manageable.

Tips for Dining Out:

1. Research the Menu: Look up the restaurant's menu online beforehand to identify carnivore-friendly options.

2. Choose the Right Restaurant: Opt for steakhouses, barbecue joints, or seafood restaurants that offer meat-centric dishes.

3. Simple Orders: Stick to plain grilled or roasted meats, and ask for butter or olive oil instead of sauces.

4. Be Clear and Confident: Politely explain your dietary needs to the server and don't hesitate to ask for modifications.

Testimonial: Mark's Dining Out Experience

Mark, who often dines out with colleagues, found that choosing the right restaurants and being clear about his dietary needs made eating out easier. "I always check the menu in advance and communicate my needs confidently. It's worked well for me," he explains.

Navigating Social Gatherings

Family Events and Parties

Social gatherings with family and friends can be tricky, especially when food is a central focus. Here are some strategies to help you navigate these events:

Tips for Social Gatherings:

1. Bring Your Own Food: Offer to bring a meat dish that you can enjoy and share with others.

2. Eat Before You Go: Have a satisfying carnivore meal before the event to avoid hunger and temptation.

3. Focus on Socializing: Shift the focus from food to enjoying conversations and activities.

4. Politely Decline: If offered foods that don't fit your diet, decline politely and explain your dietary preferences if necessary.

Testimonial: Sarah's Family Gatherings

Sarah, who follows a carnivore diet, found that bringing her own food to family gatherings helped her stay on track. "I bring a delicious meat dish that everyone enjoys, and it ensures I have something to eat," she says.

Office and Workplace Challenges

Staying on Track at Work

Navigating dietary choices in the workplace can be challenging, especially with office snacks, lunches, and social events. Here are some strategies for maintaining your carnivore diet at work:

Tips for the Workplace:

1. Prepare Your Meals: Bring your own carnivore-friendly lunches and snacks to avoid temptation.

2. Communicate with Colleagues: Explain your dietary preferences to colleagues to gain their understanding and support.

3. Stay Focused: Keep your dietary goals in mind and remember why you chose the carnivore diet.

4. Find Allies: Connect with colleagues who have similar dietary preferences or health goals.

Testimonial: John's Workplace Strategy

John, who follows a carnivore diet, found that preparing his meals and communicating with colleagues helped him stay on track. "I bring my own lunch and snacks, and my colleagues know about my diet, which makes things easier," he shares.

Managing Social Pressure

Handling Criticism and Curiosity

Social pressure and criticism are common challenges for those following a non-traditional diet. Here's how to handle these situations with confidence:

Tips for Managing Social Pressure:

1. Stay Confident: Be confident in your dietary choices and the benefits you've experienced.

2. Use Humor: Light-hearted humor can deflect criticism and ease tension.

3. Share Success Stories: Share your positive experiences and health improvements.

4. Set Boundaries: Politely but firmly set boundaries if the conversation becomes too intrusive or critical.

Testimonial: Emily's Confidence Boost

Emily, who faced criticism from friends, found that staying confident and using humor helped deflect negative comments. "I stay positive and share my success story, which usually turns the conversation around," she says.

Celebrating Special Occasions

Adapting to Holidays and Festivities

Special occasions and holidays often revolve around food, which can pose challenges for those on a carnivore diet. Here are some strategies for adapting:

Tips for Special Occasions:

1. Plan Ahead: Communicate with hosts about your dietary needs and offer to bring a carnivore-friendly dish.

2. Focus on Tradition: Enjoy the non-food aspects of the celebration, such as spending time with loved ones and participating in activities.

3. Create New Traditions: Incorporate carnivore-friendly foods into your holiday traditions.

Testimonial: David's Holiday Adaptation

David, who follows a carnivore diet, found that planning ahead and bringing his own dishes made holidays more enjoyable. "I make sure there are foods I can eat, and I focus on spending quality time with my family," he shares.

Building a Support Network

Finding Like-Minded Individuals

Having a support network of like-minded individuals can make a significant difference in your carnivore journey. Here's how to build your support network:

Tips for Building Support:

1. Join Online Communities: Participate in carnivore diet forums, social media groups, and online communities.

2. Attend Meetups: Look for local carnivore or low-carb meetups and events.

3. Connect with Friends: Reach out to friends who have similar dietary preferences or health goals.

4. Share Your Journey: Document and share your carnivore journey online to connect with others and gain support.

Testimonial: Megan's Support Network

Megan, who found support through online communities, says, "Joining carnivore diet groups online has been incredibly helpful. It's great to connect with others who share my dietary goals and experiences."

Navigating social situations on a carnivore diet may require some adjustment, but with the right strategies, you can maintain your dietary principles without sacrificing your social life. By educating friends and family, planning ahead, and building a support network, you can confidently enjoy social gatherings, dine out, and handle social pressure. Embrace the simplicity and health benefits of the carnivore diet, and remember that your well-being is worth the effort.

Chapter 12

Addressing Common Concerns

Debunking Myths and Misconceptions

As the carnivore diet gains popularity, it also attracts a fair share of myths, misconceptions, and concerns. These often stem from misunderstandings about nutrition, health, and the principles of the diet. In this chapter, we'll address common concerns and debunk myths to provide a clearer, evidence-based understanding of the carnivore diet. By dispelling these misconceptions, we aim to build confidence in the diet's efficacy and safety.

Myth 1: The Carnivore Diet Lacks Nutrients

Concern: Missing Out on Essential Vitamins and Minerals

One of the most prevalent myths is that a diet consisting solely of animal products lacks essential nutrients found in fruits, vegetables, and grains.

Fact: Animal foods are rich in a wide array of essential nutrients. Meats, especially organ meats, provide vitamins such as B12, A, D, E, and K2, as well as minerals like iron, zinc, and selenium.

Scientific Insight

Research indicates that animal-based foods offer a highly bioavailable form of many nutrients, meaning they are easier for the body to absorb and utilize compared to plant-based sources.

Testimonial: Lisa's Nutrient-Rich Diet

Lisa, who follows a strict carnivore diet, tracks her nutrient intake and has found it to be more than adequate. "Since switching to carnivore, my nutrient levels have improved, and I feel more energetic and healthier," she shares.

Myth 2: The Carnivore Diet Causes Heart Disease

Concern: High Saturated Fat and Cholesterol Intake

Many people believe that the high levels of saturated fat and cholesterol in a carnivore diet lead to heart disease.

Fact: Recent research challenges the traditional view that saturated fat and dietary cholesterol are primary causes of heart disease. Studies have shown that these nutrients can be part of a healthy diet and may not have the detrimental effects once believed.

Scientific Insight

A meta-analysis published in the American Journal of Clinical Nutrition found no significant evidence linking dietary saturated fat with an increased risk of heart disease.

Testimonial: Dr. James' Perspective

Dr. James, a cardiologist, notes, "The evidence is shifting. We see many patients with improved cardiovascular markers on low-carb and carnivore diets."

Myth 3: The Carnivore Diet Is Not Sustainable

Concern: Long-Term Adherence and Sustainability

Critics often argue that the carnivore diet is too restrictive to be sustainable in the long term.

Fact: Many individuals have successfully adhered to the carnivore diet for years, reporting sustained health benefits and satisfaction with their dietary choices. The key to sustainability is finding variety and enjoyment within the permissible foods.

Scientific Insight

Adherence to any diet is influenced by personal preference, satisfaction, and perceived benefits. The simplicity and satiety offered by the carnivore diet can enhance long-term adherence.

Testimonial: Mike's Long-Term Success

Mike, who has been following the carnivore diet for over three years, says, "I find it more sustainable than any diet I've tried. It's simple, satisfying, and I enjoy every meal."

Myth 4: The Carnivore Diet Is Harmful to Gut Health

Concern: Lack of Fiber and Gut Microbiome Impact

A common concern is that the absence of fiber in the carnivore diet negatively impacts gut health and the microbiome.

Fact: While fiber is known to benefit gut health, many individuals on a carnivore diet report significant improvements in digestive issues. The diet's anti-inflammatory properties can positively affect gut health.

Scientific Insight

Emerging research suggests that a reduction in dietary fiber can be beneficial for certain individuals with specific digestive disorders. Moreover, a carnivore diet's emphasis on nutrient-dense, easily digestible foods can support gut health.

Testimonial: Rachel's Gut Health Improvement

Rachel, who suffered from irritable bowel syndrome (IBS), found relief on the carnivore diet. "My gut health has never been better. The bloating and discomfort are gone," she says.

Myth 5: The Carnivore Diet Is Bad for the Environment

Concern: Environmental Impact of Meat Production

Environmental concerns about meat production, particularly beef, lead some to believe that a carnivore diet is environmentally unsustainable.

Fact: The environmental impact of meat production varies widely based on farming practices. Sustainable and regenerative farming methods can mitigate many of the environmental concerns associated with conventional meat production.

Scientific Insight

Regenerative agriculture, which focuses on restoring soil health and using holistic management practices, has the potential to sequester carbon and improve ecosystem health, making meat production more sustainable.

Testimonial: Sarah's Sustainable Approach

Sarah, who sources her meat from local, regenerative farms, explains, "I'm committed to supporting sustainable practices. It's possible to follow a carnivore diet and be environmentally conscious."

Myth 6: The Carnivore Diet Causes Nutritional Deficiencies

Concern: Lack of Variety Leading to Deficiencies

Some believe that the lack of dietary variety in the carnivore diet increases the risk of nutritional deficiencies.

Fact: A well-planned carnivore diet that includes a variety of meats and organ meats can provide all essential nutrients. Organ meats, in particular, are nutrient powerhouses that can prevent deficiencies.

Scientific Insight

Organ meats are among the most nutrient-dense foods available, providing vitamins, minerals, and essential fatty acids in highly bioavailable forms.

Testimonial: Alex's Nutrient Balance

Alex, who includes a range of meats and organ meats in his diet, says, "I've had my nutrient levels tested regularly, and everything is in the optimal range."

Myth 7: The Carnivore Diet Is Only for Weight Loss

Concern: Limited Health Benefits

Some people view the carnivore diet solely as a weight loss tool, doubting its broader health benefits.

Fact: Beyond weight loss, the carnivore diet has been reported to improve a range of health conditions, including autoimmune diseases, mental health disorders, and metabolic syndrome.

Scientific Insight

Case studies and anecdotal evidence suggest that the carnivore diet can have therapeutic effects on various health conditions due to its anti-inflammatory properties and nutrient density.

Testimonial: Emma's Health Transformation

Emma, who started the carnivore diet for weight loss, experienced unexpected health benefits. "I initially did it to lose weight, but my autoimmune symptoms have improved dramatically," she shares.

Myth 8: Eating Only Meat Is Boring

Concern: Lack of Culinary Variety

A common misconception is that a diet consisting only of meat is monotonous and lacks variety.

Fact: The carnivore diet can be as varied and flavorful as you make it. Different cuts of meat, cooking methods, and seasonings can provide a wide range of tastes and textures.

Scientific Insight

Culinary creativity within dietary constraints can enhance meal satisfaction and adherence. Exploring various meats and preparation techniques can keep the diet interesting.

Testimonial: Chef John's Culinary Creativity

Chef John, who follows a carnivore diet, finds joy in culinary experimentation. "I experiment with different cuts, cooking methods, and spices. It's anything but boring," he says.

Myth 9: The Carnivore Diet Is Too Expensive

Concern: High Cost of Meat

Many assume that a meat-heavy diet is prohibitively expensive.

Fact: While high-quality meats can be costly, there are strategies to keep the carnivore diet affordable, such as buying in bulk, choosing less expensive cuts, and sourcing meat locally.

Scientific Insight

Budget-friendly approaches to the carnivore diet can make it accessible to a wider audience without compromising nutritional quality.

Testimonial: David's Budget-Friendly Approach

David, who follows a carnivore diet on a budget, says, "I buy in bulk and choose cheaper cuts like ground beef and pork shoulder. It's more affordable than I expected."

Myth 10: The Carnivore Diet Is a Fad

Concern: Lack of Longevity and Research

Some view the carnivore diet as a passing trend with no scientific backing.

Fact: While research on the carnivore diet is still emerging, its principles are rooted in ancestral eating patterns. Many have experienced long-term health benefits, suggesting it's more than just a fad.

Scientific Insight

Historical and anecdotal evidence supports the idea that meat-centric diets have been a part of human evolution. Ongoing research continues to explore its health impacts.

Testimonial: Dr. Karen's Insights

Dr. Karen, a nutrition researcher, notes, "The carnivore diet is gaining attention for its potential health benefits. It's worth exploring further rather than dismissing as a fad."

Addressing common concerns and debunking myths about the carnivore diet is crucial for a clear understanding of its potential benefits and challenges. By relying on scientific evidence and real-life testimonials, we can dispel misconceptions and provide a more accurate picture of what it means to follow a carnivore diet. Armed with this knowledge, you can confidently navigate your carnivore journey, knowing you're making informed choices for your health.

Chapter 13

Advanced Tips for Long-Term Success

Maintaining Simplicity Over Time

Embracing the carnivore diet is a transformative journey that can lead to remarkable health improvements. However, maintaining this dietary lifestyle over the long term requires strategic planning, adaptation, and a focus on simplicity. In this chapter, we'll explore advanced tips and strategies for sustaining your carnivore diet for the long haul, ensuring you continue to reap its benefits while keeping your approach straightforward and enjoyable.

Prioritizing Nutrient Density

Emphasizing Quality Over Quantity

To sustain a carnivore diet, it's essential to prioritize nutrient-dense foods. Quality over quantity ensures you receive the necessary vitamins and minerals without overcomplicating your meals.

Key Strategies:

1. Choose Grass-Fed and Pasture-Raised Meats: These options tend to have higher nutrient levels, including omega-3 fatty acids and antioxidants.

2. Incorporate Organ Meats: Liver, heart, and kidneys are nutrient powerhouses that can enhance your diet.

3. Diversify Your Meat Choices: Include a variety of meats such as beef, pork, lamb, and poultry to cover a broad spectrum of nutrients.

Scientific Insight

Research shows that grass-fed and pasture-raised meats contain higher levels of beneficial nutrients like omega-3 fatty acids and conjugated linoleic acid (CLA), which support overall health.

Testimonial: Anna's Nutrient-Rich Choices

Anna, who follows a carnivore diet, emphasizes quality in her food choices. "Incorporating organ meats and grass-fed beef has made a huge difference in my health and energy levels," she says.

Simplifying Meal Preparation

Streamlining Your Cooking Routine

Keeping meal preparation simple is crucial for long-term adherence to the carnivore diet. Streamlining your cooking routine can save time and reduce stress.

Key Strategies:

1. Batch Cooking: Prepare large quantities of meat at once and store them for quick, easy meals throughout the week.
2. Use Simple Cooking Methods: Stick to grilling, baking, and slow-cooking, which are straightforward and require minimal effort.
3. Focus on Seasoning: Simple seasonings like salt, pepper, and herbs can add flavor without complicating your cooking process.

Scientific Insight

Batch cooking and simple preparation methods are associated with higher adherence to dietary plans, as they reduce the time and effort required for meal preparation.

Testimonial: Mike's Batch Cooking Routine

Mike, who has been on the carnivore diet for over two years, swears by batch cooking. "I cook a week's worth of meat on Sundays. It saves time and keeps me on track," he explains.

Monitoring Health Markers

Regular Check-Ins and Adjustments

Monitoring your health markers regularly can help you stay informed about your body's response to the diet and make necessary adjustments.

Key Strategies:

1. Regular Blood Tests: Check key markers such as cholesterol, blood sugar, and nutrient levels to ensure you're meeting your health goals.

2. Track Physical Changes: Keep a log of changes in weight, muscle mass, energy levels, and other physical indicators.

3. Listen to Your Body: Pay attention to how you feel and adjust your diet as needed based on your body's feedback.

Scientific Insight

Regular monitoring of health markers allows for timely interventions and adjustments, ensuring optimal health outcomes.

Testimonial: Dr. Laura's Approach

Dr. Laura, who follows a carnivore diet, emphasizes the importance of regular check-ins. "I get my blood work done every six months and track my energy levels daily. It helps me stay on top of my health," she says.

Staying Informed and Educated

Continuous Learning and Adaptation

Staying informed about the latest research and developments in the carnivore diet can help you make informed decisions and adapt your approach over time.

Key Strategies:

1. Read Scientific Literature: Stay updated with new studies and findings related to the carnivore diet and nutrition.

2. Join Online Communities: Engage with other carnivore diet followers to share experiences, tips, and support.

3. Consult Experts: Seek advice from nutritionists, dietitians, or doctors knowledgeable about the carnivore diet.

Scientific Insight

Continuous education and engagement with the latest research promote better dietary adherence and health outcomes.

Testimonial: Karen's Educational Journey

Karen, who has been on the carnivore diet for three years, values continuous learning. "I read research articles and participate in online forums. It keeps me informed and motivated," she shares.

Managing Social and Psychological Factors

Building a Supportive Environment

A supportive social and psychological environment is crucial for long-term success on the carnivore diet. Building a network and managing stress can enhance your adherence and well-being.

Key Strategies:

1. Find a Support Group: Join local or online support groups to connect with like-minded individuals.

2. Communicate with Loved Ones: Share your dietary journey with friends and family to gain their understanding and support.

3. Practice Stress Management: Incorporate activities like meditation, exercise, and hobbies to manage stress and maintain mental health.

Scientific Insight

Social support and effective stress management are linked to higher adherence to dietary plans and better overall health.

Testimonial: John's Support Network

John, who follows a carnivore diet, finds strength in his support network. "Having a group of people who understand and support my diet makes all the difference," he says.

Adapting to Life Changes

Flexibility and Resilience

Life is full of changes, and being flexible and resilient is key to maintaining the carnivore diet over time. Adapting to new circumstances without compromising your dietary goals is essential.

Key Strategies:

1. Plan for Travel: Research carnivore-friendly options when traveling and pack portable snacks like jerky and canned meats.

2. Adapt to New Routines: Be prepared to adjust your meal planning and cooking routines if your schedule changes.

3. Stay Positive: Embrace change with a positive mindset and view challenges as opportunities to reinforce your commitment.

Scientific Insight

Flexibility and resilience are important for sustaining long-term dietary changes, helping individuals navigate life's ups and downs without abandoning their goals.

Testimonial: Emily's Adaptability

Emily, who has maintained a carnivore diet through various life changes, says, "Flexibility has been key. I adapt my routine as needed and stay committed to my goals."

Embracing Variety within Simplicity

Exploring Culinary Creativity

Maintaining simplicity doesn't mean sacrificing variety. Exploring different cuts of meat, cooking methods, and recipes can keep your diet exciting and satisfying.

Key Strategies:

1. Experiment with New Recipes: Try new carnivore recipes to add variety to your meals.

2. Explore Different Cuts: Use various cuts of meat to introduce new flavors and textures.

3. Season Creatively: Experiment with different herbs, spices, and marinades to enhance the taste of your dishes.

Scientific Insight

Culinary creativity and variety within dietary constraints can increase satisfaction and adherence to a dietary plan.

Testimonial: Chef Lisa's Culinary Adventures

Chef Lisa, who follows a carnivore diet, enjoys experimenting in the kitchen. "I love trying new recipes and cuts of meat. It keeps my meals exciting and satisfying," she explains.

Maintaining long-term success on the carnivore diet involves strategic planning, continuous learning, and a focus on simplicity. By prioritizing nutrient density, simplifying meal preparation, monitoring health markers, staying informed, managing social and psychological factors, adapting to life changes, and embracing variety within simplicity, you can sustain this dietary lifestyle and continue to enjoy its numerous health benefits. Embrace the journey with confidence and commitment, knowing that your efforts will lead to a healthier, more vibrant life.

Chapter 14

The Carnivore Diet for Families

Adapting the Diet for All Ages

The carnivore diet, while often discussed in the context of individual health transformations, can be a beneficial lifestyle for families as well. Adapting the carnivore diet for all ages, from children to seniors, requires thoughtful planning and consideration of each family member's unique nutritional needs. This chapter will explore how to implement the carnivore diet within a family setting, ensuring that everyone can enjoy its benefits safely and effectively.

Understanding Nutritional Needs Across Life Stages

Infants and Toddlers

For the youngest family members, nutrition is critical for growth and development. While the carnivore diet can be adapted for older children, infants and toddlers have specific nutritional needs that must be met.

Key Strategies:

1. Breastfeeding: Breast milk or formula should be the primary source of nutrition for infants up to one year.

2. Introducing Solid Foods: Begin with nutrient-dense animal foods like pureed meats, bone broths, and soft-cooked egg yolks as infants transition to solids.

3. Monitoring Growth: Regular check-ups with a pediatrician are essential to ensure that infants and toddlers are meeting their growth milestones.

Scientific Insight

Breast milk provides essential nutrients tailored to an infant's needs. Introducing nutrient-dense animal foods can support growth and development as infants transition to solid foods.

Testimonial: Emily's Experience

Emily, a mother of two, introduced her children to nutrient-dense animal foods early on. "My kids thrived on pureed liver and bone broths. They're healthy and growing well," she shares.

Children and Adolescents

As children grow, their nutritional needs change. A carnivore diet can support their development, but it's important to ensure they receive a balanced intake of essential nutrients.

Key Strategies:

1. Variety of Meats: Offer a range of meats, including beef, pork, poultry, and fish, to provide diverse nutrients.

2. Incorporate Organ Meats: Include nutrient-rich organ meats in meals to enhance vitamin and mineral intake.

3. Educational Involvement: Involve children in meal planning and preparation to foster an understanding of healthy eating habits.

Scientific Insight

A varied diet rich in animal proteins and fats supports physical and cognitive development in children and adolescents.

Testimonial: Lisa's Approach

Lisa, a mother of three, emphasizes variety in her children's diet. "We eat different types of meat and organs. The kids are energetic and perform well in school," she notes.

Adults

For adults, the carnivore diet can offer numerous health benefits, from weight management to improved mental clarity. Tailoring the diet to individual needs and lifestyles is key.

Key Strategies:

1. Focus on Nutrient Density: Choose high-quality, nutrient-dense meats to maximize health benefits.
2. Meal Planning: Develop a consistent meal planning routine to simplify daily eating and ensure nutrient intake.
3. Listen to Your Body: Pay attention to hunger and satiety signals to maintain a balanced diet.

Scientific Insight

A diet rich in animal-based nutrients can support overall health, including muscle maintenance, cognitive function, and metabolic health.

Testimonial: John's Routine

John, who follows the carnivore diet, finds it straightforward and effective. "I feel more focused and energetic. Planning my meals helps me stay on track," he explains.

Seniors

Older adults have unique nutritional requirements, and a carnivore diet can support healthy aging. Focusing on easy-to-digest, nutrient-rich foods is important.

Key Strategies:

1. Soft and Easy-to-Chew Foods: Incorporate softer meats and broths to accommodate dental issues or digestive sensitivities.

2. Bone Broths: Include bone broths for their collagen and mineral content, which support joint health and digestion.

3. Monitor Nutrient Intake: Regularly check nutrient levels, particularly vitamin B12, iron, and calcium, to ensure adequate intake.

Scientific Insight

Nutrient-dense, easily digestible foods can help seniors maintain muscle mass, bone health, and overall vitality.

Testimonial: Margaret's Diet

Margaret, a senior on the carnivore diet, enjoys its simplicity. "I eat a lot of soft-cooked meats and broths. My digestion is better, and I feel more energetic," she says.

Practical Tips for Family Implementation
Meal Planning and Preparation

Efficient meal planning and preparation can help integrate the carnivore diet into a busy family lifestyle.

Key Strategies:

1. Batch Cooking: Prepare large quantities of meats and broths that can be easily reheated for quick meals.

2. Family Favorites: Identify and rotate family-favorite recipes to keep meals enjoyable and varied.

3. Involve Everyone: Encourage family members to participate in meal preparation to foster teamwork and make cooking a fun activity.

Scientific Insight

Family involvement in meal planning and preparation can improve dietary adherence and satisfaction, creating positive eating habits.

Testimonial: The Thompson Family

The Thompson family enjoys cooking together. "We batch cook on weekends, and everyone helps out. It makes mealtime more enjoyable," says Mr. Thompson.

Addressing Picky Eaters

Children and even some adults can be picky eaters. Finding ways to make meat appealing and palatable is crucial for adherence.

Key Strategies:

1. Creative Presentation: Use fun shapes, skewers, and presentation techniques to make meat more appealing to children.

2. Flavor Variety: Experiment with different seasonings and marinades to add variety and enhance flavors.

3. Consistency: Offer new foods consistently, as repeated exposure can help develop a taste for them.

Scientific Insight

Repeated exposure to new foods can increase acceptance, particularly in children. Creative presentation and variety in flavors can make meals more appealing.

Testimonial: Sarah's Success with Picky Eaters

Sarah, a mother of two picky eaters, shares, "I use cookie cutters to shape meat and add different herbs and spices. The kids are more willing to try new things now."

Navigating Social Situations

Eating out and attending social events can be challenging on a carnivore diet. Planning and flexibility are key to navigating these situations.

Key Strategies:

1. Plan Ahead: Research restaurant menus in advance to find carnivore-friendly options.

2. Bring Your Own: When attending social events, bring your own carnivore-friendly dishes to ensure you have suitable food.

3. Communicate: Inform hosts or friends about your dietary preferences to avoid surprises and ensure there are options available.

Scientific Insight

Planning and clear communication can help manage social dining experiences and maintain dietary adherence.

Testimonial: Emma's Social Strategy

Emma, who follows a carnivore diet, always plans ahead. "I check menus online and often bring my own dish to parties. It makes socializing easier and stress-free," she says.

Family Health and Well-Being

Monitoring Health Markers

Regular health check-ups and monitoring can ensure that all family members are thriving on the carnivore diet.

Key Strategies:

1. Regular Check-Ups: Schedule periodic health check-ups for the entire family to monitor growth, development, and overall health.

2. Nutrient Testing: Conduct regular blood tests to check for any potential deficiencies and adjust the diet accordingly.

3. Health Journals: Maintain health journals for each family member to track physical and mental health changes and dietary responses.

Scientific Insight

Regular monitoring and adjustments based on health markers can help maintain optimal health and address any emerging issues promptly.

Testimonial: The Miller Family's Approach

The Miller family keeps health journals for each member. "We track our health and make dietary adjustments as needed. It keeps us all in great shape," says Mrs. Miller.

Adapting the carnivore diet for families involves understanding the unique nutritional needs of each family member and implementing practical strategies to ensure long-term success. By focusing on nutrient density, simplifying meal preparation, involving everyone in the process, and monitoring health markers, families can thrive on the carnivore diet. Embrace the journey together, knowing that you are fostering a healthy, sustainable lifestyle for your entire family.

Conclusion

Living a Pure Carnivore Lifestyle for Optimal Health

The journey of embracing a pure carnivore lifestyle is not just a dietary shift but a profound transformation that impacts every facet of life. As we conclude this exploration into simplifying your diet and amplifying your health, it's essential to reflect on the core principles that make the carnivore diet both a powerful and sustainable choice.

Embracing Simplicity and Clarity

The Power of Simplification

In a world filled with dietary complexities and conflicting nutritional advice, the carnivore diet stands out for its simplicity. By focusing solely on nutrient-dense animal foods, you strip away the confusion and embrace a clear, straightforward approach to eating.

Key Takeaways:

1. Eliminate Dietary Noise: Removing processed foods, sugars, and plant-based toxins can lead to significant health improvements.

2. Focus on Quality: Prioritizing high-quality, nutrient-dense meats ensures that you receive the essential vitamins and minerals your body needs.

3. Enjoy Mental Clarity: Simplifying your diet can reduce decision fatigue, leading to enhanced mental clarity and focus.

Testimonial: David's Clarity

David found that simplifying his diet improved his mental health. "I no longer worry about what to eat. My mind feels clearer and more focused," he says.

Achieving Optimal Health

The Comprehensive Benefits

Throughout this book, we've explored the numerous health benefits of a carnivore diet. From weight loss and muscle gain to improved mental clarity and better digestion, the advantages are compelling and well-documented.

Key Takeaways:

1. Sustained Energy Levels: A meat-only diet provides consistent energy without the crashes associated with carbohydrate consumption.

2. Enhanced Physical Performance: Increased protein intake supports muscle growth, recovery, and overall physical performance.

3. Improved Mental Health: The carnivore diet's impact on brain health can lead to better mood stability, reduced anxiety, and enhanced cognitive function.

Testimonial: Rachel's Transformation

Rachel experienced a dramatic health transformation. "I have more energy, my mood is stable, and I feel stronger than ever," she shares.

Overcoming Challenges

Navigating Potential Obstacles

Every dietary change comes with challenges, but the carnivore diet's simplicity makes it easier to navigate potential obstacles. By addressing common concerns and adopting practical strategies, you can overcome these challenges and stay committed to your health journey.

Key Takeaways:

1. Social Situations: Plan ahead for dining out and social gatherings to ensure you have carnivore-friendly options.

2. Meal Preparation: Simplify your cooking routine with batch cooking and easy-to-prepare meals.

3. Long-Term Sustainability: Focus on nutrient density, regular health monitoring, and continuous learning to sustain your diet over time.

Testimonial: Mark's Success

Mark navigated social challenges by planning ahead. "I always have a plan for social events. It keeps me on track and reduces stress," he notes.

Building a Supportive Environment

Fostering Family and Community Support

A successful dietary lifestyle often depends on a supportive environment. Whether it's involving your family in meal planning or connecting with like-minded individuals online, building a support network is crucial.

Key Takeaways:

1. Family Involvement: Encourage family participation in meal planning and preparation to create a unified approach to health.

2. Online Communities: Join online forums and social media groups to share experiences, gain insights, and find encouragement.

3. Educational Resources: Stay informed through continuous learning and consultation with experts to enhance your dietary knowledge.

Testimonial: The Johnson Family's Unity

The Johnson family embraced the carnivore diet together. "We support each other and learn together. It's brought us closer as a family," says Mrs. Johnson.

The Long-Term Vision

Looking Ahead to a Healthier Future

Adopting a pure carnivore lifestyle is not just a short-term diet but a long-term commitment to optimal health. By embracing simplicity, focusing on nutrient density, and building a supportive environment, you set the stage for lasting health and well-being.

Key Takeaways:

1. Sustainability: Focus on long-term strategies that make the diet easy to maintain and enjoyable.

2. Adaptability: Be flexible and ready to adapt your approach as needed to fit different life stages and circumstances.

3. Commitment: Stay committed to your health goals, knowing that the benefits of the carnivore diet will continue to unfold over time.

Testimonial: Jane's Long-Term Success

Jane has sustained her carnivore lifestyle for years. "I've never felt better. The simplicity and benefits keep me committed," she explains.

Living a pure carnivore lifestyle is a powerful way to achieve optimal health. By simplifying your diet, focusing on quality nutrition, and building a supportive environment, you can enjoy sustained energy, enhanced mental clarity, and overall well-being. Embrace the journey with confidence, knowing that you are making a positive, lasting impact on your health and the health of your family. The carnivore diet is more than just a way of eating; it's a pathway to a healthier, happier life.

www.ingramcontent.com/pod-product-compliance
Lightning Source LLC
Chambersburg PA
CBHW071012250726
48653CB00005B/1593